Skin T

Natural DIY Methods of removing Mole, Wart

and Skin Tag

Singe Lamett

ISBN: 978-1-63750-257-0

Table of Contents

SKIN TAG 1

INTRODUCTION 4

CHAPTER 1...7

HOW TO IDENTIFY PORES AND SKIN TAG 7

WHAT CAUSES PORES AND SKIN TAGS 8

When to see a Medical Expert..............................10

HOW TO REMOVE PORES AND SKIN TAGS...........................11

SKIN TAG ON EYELID REMOVAL 13

Preventing pores and skin tags 19

TREATMENT 20

CHAPTER 2...24

WHY DOES SKIN TAG OCCUR..24

Removing pores and skin tags..............................25

CHAPTER 3...28

HOME REMEDY FOR SKIN TAG REMOVAL...........................28

WHEN TO SEE A MEDICAL EXPERT 35

CHAPTER 4...36

TOOTHPASTE FOR SKIN TAG REMOVAL 36

WILL TOOTHPASTE HARM MY SKIN? 39

HOW LONG DOES IT TAKE FOR PORES AND SKIN TAG TO FALL OFF?................................41

CHAPTER 5...45

4 DIY SKIN TAG REMOVER METHODS 45

ì

Introduction

Epidermis/skin tags are flesh-colored growths that form on the skin's surface; they suspend from a thin piece of tissues called a stalk. These growths are common, and about 25% of trusted sources of individuals have at least one epidermis/skin tag.

You'll usually find pores and skin tags in folds of the epidermis/skin in these areas:

- Armpits.

- Neck.

- Under the breasts.

- Round the genitals.

Pores and skin tags are painless, non-cancerous growths on your skin; they're linked to your skin by a little, slim stalk called a *peduncle*. Epidermis/skin tags are regular in men and women, especially after age group 50; they can show up anywhere on the body, though they're common within places where your skin layer folds like the:

- Armpits.

- Groin.

- Thighs.

- Eyelids.

- Neck.

- Area under your breasts.

Less often, pores and skin tags can grow on the eyelids. Pores and skin tags don't cause any health issues; however, they can be unpleasant if indeed they rub against your clothes, and you will possibly not like how they look.

After reading this book, you will be glad you did and would have learnt what you should know to remove your skin tag and wheat to avoid.

Chapter 1

How to identify Pores and Skin tag

The primary way to recognize a skin tag is by the peduncle; unlike moles plus some other pores and skin growths, epidermis/skin tags suspend off your skin by this small stalk.

Most pores and skin tags are small, typically smaller than 2 millimetres in proportions; some can develop as large as several centimetres. Pores and skin tags are smooth touches. They might be natural and circular, or they might be wrinkly and asymmetrical. Some epidermis/skin tags are threadlike and resemble grains of grain.

Epidermis/skin tags may be flesh-colored; they may also be darker than the encompassing skin credited to *hyperpigmentation*. If an epidermis/skin tag becomes twisted, it could turn black credited too little blood flow.

What causes pores and skin tags

It's unclear what exactly causes epidermis/skin tags. Given that they usually arrive in pores and skin folds, friction may are likely involved. Skin tags are made of arteries and collagen surrounded by an external layer of the epidermis/skin.

Relating to a 2008 research, the human being papillomavirus (HPV) may be considered a factor in the introduction of pores and skin tags. The analysis analyzed 37 epidermis/skin tags from various sites of your body. Results demonstrated HPV DNA in almost 50 percent of your skin tags examined.

Insulin resistance, which might lead to type 2 diabetes and prediabetes, could also are likely involved in the introduction of pores and skin tags. People who have an insulin level of resistance don't absorb blood sugar effectively from the bloodstream. Regarding a 2010 research, the existence of multiple epidermis/skin tags was associated with insulin level of resistance, *a higher body mass index, and high triglycerides.*

Pores and skin tags are also a common side-effect of pregnancy; this can be due to being pregnant hormones and putting on weight. In rare circumstances, multiple pores and skin tags can be considered a sign of the hormone imbalance or an endocrine problem.

Epidermis/skin tags aren't contagious; there could be a hereditary connection. It isn't uncommon for multiple families to keep these things.

Risky things to consider

You might be at a higher threat of getting skin tags if you:

- Are overweight

- Are pregnant

- Have family who has epidermis/skin tags

- Have insulin resistance or type 2 diabetes

- Have HPV

Pores and skin tags don't become pores and skin cancer. Irritation might occur if indeed they rub with clothing, jewellery, or another epidermis/skin. Shave with caution around pores and skin tags.

Shaving off pores and skin tag won't cause long term damage, though it could distress and prolonged blood loss.

When to see a Medical Expert

Since some moles may be cancerous, it's better to have

your skin layer tags analyzed by a health care provider; other skin conditions such as warts and moles can resemble skin tags. Your doctor can diagnose epidermis/skin tags. They'll likely do that through a visible exam. If indeed they have any questions about the analysis, they could also execute a biopsy.

How to remove Pores and Skin Tags

Tiny skin tags may rub off independently; however, most epidermis/skin tags stay mounted on your skin. Generally, pores and skin tags don't require treatment, if epidermis/skin tags harm or frustrate you, you may choose to keep these things removed.

Your physician may remove your skin layer tags by:

- ***Cryotherapy:*** Freezing your skin tag with liquid nitrogen.

- ***Surgery:*** Removing your skin tag with scissors or a scalpel.

- ***Electrosurgery:*** Burning away the skin tag with high-frequency electricity.

- ***Ligation:*** Removing your skin tag by tying it off with surgical thread to be able to take off its blood circulation.

Having small pores and skin tags removed doesn't usually require anaesthesia, your physician could use local anaesthesia when eliminating large or multiple pores and skin tags; you can even try natural treatments to eliminate skin tags *(Included in these are tea tree essential oil, apple cider vinegar, and lemon juice)*. Take into account that there's no medical evidence to aid these remedies.

It's will's idea to attempt to remove epidermis/skin tags by yourself; several articles offer DIY instructions for getting rid of pores and skin tags by tying them off with string or applying a chemical substance peel off, which is not very ideal and recommended. Even in a sterile environment, eliminating epidermis/skin tags could cause blood loss, burns, and contamination. It's better to let your physician handle the work.

Skin tag on eyelid removal

You don't have to eliminate a skin tag unless it bothers you. If you'd like to remove pores and skin tags for aesthetic reasons, you have a few options.

At-home treatments

Some websites recommend using home cures like apple cider vinegar to eliminate epidermis/skin tags. However, before you try removing a skin tag yourself using apple cider vinegar, consult with your skin doctor. You don't want to injure your very delicate eye area.

If your skin layer tag has a fragile base, you may be in a position to tie it off at the bottom with a bit of dental care floss or cotton; this will take off its blood circulation. Eventually, your skin tag will fall off. Ask a health care provider again before trying this technique. Removing pores and skin tags with a solid base might lead to a great deal of blood loss or contamination. You could also leave scar tissue on your eyelid.

Surgical procedure and treatments

You're safest leaving pores and skin tag removal to a skin doctor, which is one of the techniques a health care provider will use to eliminate the extra little bit of epidermis/skin from your eyelid; this treatment will remedy the skin tags you have, and yet they won't prevent new pores and skin tags from showing up in the foreseeable future.

Cryotherapy

Cryotherapy uses extreme chilly to freeze off epidermis/skin tags; your physician will apply water nitrogen to your skin layer on the cotton swab, or with a set of tweezers. The liquid may sting or burn off a little when it continues on your skin layer; the frozen pores and the skin tag will fall off within ten times.

A blister will form in the region where the water nitrogen was applied, which should scab over and fall off within two weeks to a month.

Surgical removal

Another way to eliminate skin tags is to trim them off.

Your physician will first numb the region, and then take

off the skin tag with a scalpel or special medical scissors.

Electrosurgery

Electrosurgery uses warmth to melt away the skin tag at the bottom. Burning prevents excessive blood loss when the tag is removed.

Ligation

Throughout a ligation procedure, a health care provider ties off underneath of your skin tag to take off its blood circulation. After a week or two, the skin tag will perish and fall off.

What causes epidermis/skin tags on eyelids?

Skin tags are produced from a protein called *collagen and arteries*, surrounded by a layer of pores and skin; doctors don't know precisely what causes them because you'll usually find tags in epidermis/skin folds like your armpits, groin, or eyelids, friction from pores and skin rubbing against epidermis/skin may be engaged.

Folks who are overweight or obese will get pores and skin tags because they have extra epidermis/skin folds. Hormone changes during pregnancy can also raise the likelihood of epidermis/skin tags forming; there could be a connection between insulin resistance, diabetes, and pores and skin tags.

People tend to get more epidermis/skin tags as they age; these growths often pop-up in middle age group and beyond. Epidermis/skin tags may run in the family; it's possible that one person inherits an elevated probability of getting these pores and skin growths.

Preventing pores and skin tags

It's impossible to avoid every skin tag, and you can lessen your probability of getting them by maintaining at a wholesome weight. Below are a few prevention tips:

- Work with your physician and a dietitian to plan foods that are lower in saturated body fat and calories.

- Exercise at medium or high strength for at least thirty minutes each day, five times a week.

- Keep all epidermis/skin folds dry to avoid friction; pat your skin layer completely dry once you shower. Apply baby natural powder to pores and skin folds like your underarms that tend to trap moisture.

- Don't wear clothing or jewelry that irritates your

skin layer. Choose soft, breathable materials like cotton rather than nylon or spandex.

Risk to consider

You're much more likely to get epidermis/skin tags if you:

- Are overweight or obese.

- Are pregnant.

- Have type 2 diabetes.

- Are in your 40s or older.

- Have other families with pores and skin tags.

Treatment

As pores and skin tags are usually safe, removal is generally for visual or aesthetic reasons. Large epidermis/skin tags, especially in areas where they could rub against something, such as clothing, jewelry or pores, and skin, may be removed credited to irritation.

Removing a big skin tag from the facial skin or under the hands can make shaving easier.

Surgery

The following methods can be utilized:

- *Cauterization*: Your skin tag is burned up using electrolysis.

- *Cryosurgery*: Your skin tag is frozen off utilizing a probe containing water nitrogen.

- *Ligation*: The blood circulation to your skin tag is interrupted.

- *Excision*: The tag is slice out with a scalpel.

These methods should only be achieved with a dermatologist, or specialist health-care professional, or a similarly trained medical expert. Epidermis/skin tags on the eyelid, especially those near to the eyelid margin, may need to be removed by an ophthalmologist, or specialist vision doctor.

Removing pores and skin tag at home is not frequently suggested, thanks to a threat of blood loss and possible infection. However, small tags can be removed by tying dental floss or little cotton thread around the bottom of the tag to take off blood circulation to the tag.

Over-the-counter solutions

Over-the-counter (OTC) solutions can be found at

pharmacies; these freeze your skin tag, and it'll fall off after 7 to 10 times, which can also be purchased online, though it is preferred that healthcare advice is gotten before using these treatments. These medications act like those used for wart removal; no evidence removing skin tags encourages more of these to develop.

Chapter 2

Why does Skin Tag Occur

Skin tags are made of loose collagen fibers and arteries surrounded by pores and skin. Collagen is a kind of protein found throughout your body. Men and women can have skin tags; they tend to happen in the elderly and folks who are obese or have type 2 diabetes.

Pregnant women can also be much more likely to build up skin tags consequently of changes in their hormone levels. Some individuals develop them for no apparent reason. Skin tags tend to grow in your skin folds, where the epidermis/skin rubs against itself, such as on the neck, armpits or groin. That is why they tend to affect obese individuals who have extra folds of pores and tags and epidermis/skin chafing.

When pores and skin tags can be considered a problem

Pores and skin tags are harmless and don't usually distress or discomfort. However, you might consider having epidermis/skin tags removed if they are affecting your self-confidence, or if indeed they snag on clothing or jewellery and bleed; you'll usually need to pay to have this done privately. It is because skin tag removal is undoubtedly plastic surgery, which is rarely available through the NHS; plastic surgery is usually only on the NHS if the problem has effects on your physical or mental health. Sometimes, pores and skin tags fall off independently if the cells have twisted and died from too little blood supply.

Removing pores and skin tags

Do not make an effort to remove an epidermis/skin tag without talking with your doctor first. When you have pores and skin tag that's leading to problems, consider making a scheduled appointment with a privately practicing GP to get it removed. Skin tags can be burnt or frozen off similarly to how warts are removed; they may also be surgically removed, sometimes using a local anesthetic.

Freezing or burning up pores and skin tags can cause irritation and short-term pores and skin discoloration, and your skin tag might not fall off, and additional treatment may be needed.

Surgical removal gets the benefit of obliterating your skin tag, but there's a risk of small bleeding. If your skin layer tag is small with a narrow base, your GP may claim that you make an effort to take it off yourself; for example, they could suggest tying off the bottom of your skin tag with dental care floss or cotton to take off its blood circulation and make it fall off (ligation); never try to remove large epidermis/skin tags yourself because they'll bleed severely.

Chapter 3

Home Remedy for Skin tag removal

Consult a medical practitioner before trying the following methods.

1. *A tag removal device*

Home remedies are for sale to skin tag removal, you can purchase online and in many stores; however, epidermis/skin tags do not require treatment and could fall away independently, but medical removal is available.

People use these devices as a medium to obtain blood to the bottom of the tag with a little band; the medical community identifies this technique as ligation, and without a way to obtain blood, the cells will die, and the tag will drop away, usually within ten days.

2. *String*

Some people make an effort to achieve ligation with a bit of oral floss or string, which could be tricky to get this done with no help of the device or someone else because when the blood circulation has been taken off for at least a couple of days, the tag should fall away; it might be necessary to tighten up the string or floss every day.

Ensure you take the precaution of cleaning your skin, string, and hands thoroughly to avoid infection.

3. *Skin tag removal cream*

Packages containing cream and an applicator can be found in pharmacies. Instructions for some packages recommend cleaning your skin with alcoholic wipes and processing down the tag before applying the cream, to ensure that it's fully absorbed.

The cream could cause a mild stinging sensation; however, tags should fall off within 2-3 weeks.

4. *Freezing kit*

An individual can use something containing liquid nitrogen to freeze off skin tags; the products tend to be available in drugstores and pharmacies. Ensure you follow instructions because several applications may be necessary before a tag falls away, but this usually occurs within ten times.

The spray shouldn't touch surrounding pores and skin, but a person may choose to apply vaseline to the region around the tag for protection.

5. *Tea tree oil*

Tea tree oil can be a gas used to take care of several pores and skin conditions, including epidermis/skin tags.

People typically apply a few drops of the essential oil to a cotton ball, that they then affix to your skin tag with a bandage; the cotton ball is usually left on your skin layer for ten minutes, 3 times daily. It might take several times or weeks for the tag to fall off.

This treatment should be utilized with caution, as tea tree oil may irritate sensitive skin. Never use tea tree essential oil for tags located around the eyes.

6. *Apple cider vinegar*

Little research has been conducted on the potency of apple cider vinegar for pores and skin tag removal; people often soak a cotton ball in the vinegar and affix it to the tag with a bandage for ten minutes several times each day, until the tag falls away.

7. _Iodine_

Anecdotal evidence shows that an individual can use liquid iodine to eliminate skin tags.

First,

- Protect the encompassing skin through the use of vaseline or coconut essential oil to the region.

- Soak a Q-tip in iodine and pass on the liquid over the tag.

- Cover the area with a bandage before iodine has dried out.

Continue doing this treatment twice per day until the tag drops off.

8. _Cutting_

A health care provider may recommend trimming away

the development with a clean knife or scissors; never attempt this with medium or large pores and skin tags, as this may cause blood loss. Tags usually measure from a few millimetres to 2 inches in width.

Only think about this method if your skin tag has a fragile base; however, scissors and cutting blades should be sterilized before and after use. It is also essential to seek expert advice before attempting this technique, and not cut off epidermis/skin tags located throughout the eye or genitals.

Home remedies aren't suitable for pores and skin tags that are:

- Located close to the eyes.

- Located at the genitals.

- Very large or long.

- Causing pain, blood loss, or itching.

Seek treatment in such cases. Listed below are medical ways of skin tag removal:

- Cauterization: This calls for burning off your skin tag. Most tags will drop away after a couple of treatments.

- Cryotherapy: A medical expert will apply liquid nitrogen to freeze from the tag. Usually, a couple of treatments will be sufficient.

- Ligation: The tag is linked off with surgical thread, to lessen blood flow.

- Excision: A specialist use a knife to take off the tag.

Skin tag removal is usually considered beauty, which is

unlikely to be included in health insurance.

When to see a medical expert

If epidermis/skin tags that are large, painful, or situated in delicate areas, such a person should see a medical expert.

Seek prompt treatment if an epidermis/skin tag:

- Bleeds.

- Itches.

- changes form or appearance.

Chapter 4

Toothpaste for Skin Tag Removal

Toothpaste was not developed to take care of pores and skin tags; however, this will not imply that toothpaste cannot remove your skin layer tags, toothpaste will most likely contain hydrogen peroxide to assist in the whole tooth whitening process. Hydrogen peroxide will more than simply pearly white teeth though; besides, it dries out your skin.

Drying out your skin is precisely what you must do to remove pores and skin tags; which means that applying toothpaste which has hydrogen peroxide to your skin layer tags will eventually make your skin layer tags dry and fall off. However, you may still find some things that you need to know before grabbing the toothpaste from your medication cupboard and rubbing it on your skin layer tags.

Can I use any Toothpaste?

The one first thing you need to know is the kind of toothpaste that you'll need to use to eliminate a skin tag; you cannot just use any toothpaste and expect excellent results.

First,

- *The toothpaste must contain hydrogen peroxide*: Toothpaste which has hydrogen peroxide is often sold as *"whitening toothpaste"* or something such as that. Just look for hydrogen peroxide on the ingredient list.

- *Not all toothpaste is established equivalent*: Many kinds of toothpaste are created from gel because which makes them simpler to use. Gel toothpaste will most likely taste much better than regular toothpaste since it consists of artificial tastes. These artificial tastes might have great flavor and make cleaning your tooth bearable; however, they can appeal to ants and could have a reduced impact on your skin. More importantly, they are doing nothing at all to help remove epidermis/skin tags.

For both listed reasons, you should use an ordinary white toothpaste (not gel) which has hydrogen peroxide when putting it on to your skin layer tags; this will boost the effectiveness and reduce the potential for any unwanted effects, and this kind of toothpaste also will cost significantly less than gel-based toothpaste.

Will Toothpaste harm my Skin?

Toothpaste contains hydrogen peroxide which will dry out your skin; which means that utilizing it helps to treat pores, skin tags, and cause lines and wrinkles. Fortunately, there is no need to use the toothpaste to your skin layer to remove your skin tag; you can easily apply the toothpaste to only your skin tag carefully; this will reduce the unwanted effects of your skin toothpaste on your skin layer.

It's also advisable to use toothpaste (not gel) which has hydrogen peroxide no artificial flavors as stated earlier.

How exactly to Use Toothpaste on Pores and skin

- Put a little amount of toothpaste on your finger and then rub everything over your skin layer tag.

- Do not get any toothpaste on your skin layer since it will dry your skin layer and cause lines and wrinkles.

- Do not be concerned if you get just a little toothpaste on your skin layer; use a washcloth with lukewarm water and wipe away the surplus toothpaste.

Many people prefer to place a band-aid on the skin tag after applying the toothpaste; doing this is not a necessary step, but it additionally won't have any adverse effect on your skin layer. Instead, it'll keep carefully the toothpaste set up and can prevent it from being wiped away.

Also, many people prefer to use toothpaste with lukewarm water before each goes to sleep. This choice is your decision. If you applied the toothpaste and then your skin tag, then you certainly do not need to eliminate it before sleep.

How long does it take for pores and skin tag to fall off?

The amount of time it requires for your skin tag to fall off depends on a few factors, including how frequently you apply the toothpaste to your skin layer tag and how big is your skin layer tag. A standard sized skin tag, for example, should take in regards to a week to fall off if you regularly apply toothpaste to it; this consists of applying before going to sleep and soon after you awaken. It's also advisable to use it every few hours and once you have a shower.

The progress will be slow initially, but it will eventually dry and fall off with plenty of time, so don't get thrilled when it starts to pass away and rip it out. You want to buy to fall off generally as this will ensure that the whole skin tag is dead and can not reappear. Do not pick and choose at your skin tag, nor draw it off yourself.

Applying a band-aid to your skin tag may or might not help; it can tend to dry the tag a bit more, however, the fact that toothpaste requires a somewhat very long time to remove your skin tag might be slightly irritating. People usually want to see instant results; however, for this solution to work, you'll need patience.

Additionally, immediately removing skin tags often leads to permanent scars; you merely have to weigh the advantages of quickly getting rid of the skin tag and using a permanent (small) scar tissue versus eliminating the skin tag over weekly and having no scar tissue.

Final Thoughts

Toothpaste for epidermis/skin tag removal is an excellent choice for anybody that wants to make use of more natural treatments to eliminate a skin tag. Also, it effectively reduces the chance of scarring, and it's a way that doesn't involve needing to use any over-the-counter products you are uncertain of. You merely have to give it time for you to work.

You need to be careful never to get too much toothpaste on your skin layer. The hydrogen peroxide will dry your skin layer, which can result in wrinkles. Also, you will need to make sure that the growths are just pores and skin tags. If you're uncertain, you should seek assistance from your skin doctor to eliminate any other epidermis/skin conditions that can be more serious.

Other natural treatments include apple cider vinegar and the utilization of tea tree oil with coconut oil if you are thinking about alternative skin tag removal methods. Your skin doctor can help show you through your alternatives and answer any questions you might have.

Chapter 5

4 DIY Skin Tag Remover Methods

So you've decided that your skin layer tag is bothering you; As long as the tag is not infected or near a delicate area, you can address it yourself at home. Below, you will find four (4) of the highest skin tag removal methods that you can test in the comfort and confines of your home; the 4th method is not suggested for home use, though many still try to check it out despite its risks.

- Tie your skin tag off

- Use Wart Remover

- Try Essential Oils

- Scratch the tag off

Let's check out each one of these methods for pores and

skin tag removal comprehensive.

METHOD #1: *Tying your skin tag off*

Tying pores and skin tags off is a preferred solution to remove pores and skin tags in a medical office; until lately there weren't many choices available to do that quickly and securely at home. You will find devices that do that for you which prevent infection; a favourite tool that will do this for you is the *Tagband Device*; with this product that will come in pores and skin tag removal package, you can certainly get rid of your skin layer tags at home. Before this device was available, people used *dental floss or sewing thread* as a chance to skin tag removal method. However, both these methods do leave the region prone to illness. Plus, because sewing thread is so razor-sharp, it can leave the region more injured and sore. The discomfort may lead to higher chance of disease.

Ways to get rid of epidermis/skin tags by tying them off

Proper Analysis: Always be sure you check with a health care provider or dermatologist to ensure that the development is an epidermis/skin tag rather than a wart or another thing that may be more serious.

Clean the region: Use cleaning soap and drinking water on the region; then pat it dried out and dab on massaging alcoholic beverages to sterilize it.

Find the Stalk: Be sure you are apparent on what area to connect off.

Wrap Dental care Floss Around the bottom of the Stalk: Connect it securely so that it stops blood circulation; however, not so limited that it slashes into your skin layer.

Sterilize the region Daily: Keep the area carefully clean and protect it with a bandage; check the region daily and apply alcoholic beverages or antibiotic cream to keep it from getting contaminated.

Wait in regards to a Week: Your skin tag should fall off during this period.

Benefits of Tying a Pores and skin Tag Off

- You can do it at home.

- You merely need teeth floss, rubbing alcohol, and bandages.

- It's simple enough.

- It ought to be almost painless.

- It's the easiest skin tag removal method.

Negatives of Tying an Epidermis/skin Tag Off

- It could cause irritation.

- You shouldn't get it done on sensitive areas or near your groin.

- You can get an infection.

METHOD #2: Use Wart Remover

Some wart removers also focus on pores and skin tags; the ones that do, often are certain to get past them with just one single use. Though not a clinically proven method on epidermis/skin tag removal, most wart removers contain salicylic acidity or other elements.

Anecdotal evidence works with salicylic acidity as highly effective pores and skin tag remover.

Other wart removers contain water nitrogen; this is the same material that doctors use to freeze off epidermis/skin tags; if you are using something like nitrogen in it, the tag will eventually change colors and fall off. Some wart removers market themselves as pores and skin tag removers; those generally include an entire kit, filled with cream and applicator.

Ways to get Gone Skin Tags Using Wart Remover

Proper Diagnosis: Be confident the region you are dealing with is pores and skin tags.

Clean the region: Use cleaning soap and drinking water then pat dried out.

Apply Cream: Be sure you follow instructions on the bundle. Most recommend having the cream on for about 20 minutes.

Wash and Pat Dry out: Rinse the region with drinking water to thoroughly take away the cream. Pat dried out gently.

Keep the Area Clean carefully and Guarded: A little scab will form post-treatment. Keep the crust carefully clean and guarded until it falls off about three weeks later.

Advantages of Wart Remover to eliminate Skin Tags

- It's pretty inexpensive.

- It's fast and simple.

- One treatment may look after them.

Disadvantages of Wart Remover to eliminate Skin Tags

- It could sting when you are using the procedure.

- Redness might occur afterward.

- All wart removers are developed differently, and that means you might not find one which works for you immediately.

METHOD #3: Try Essential Natural oils for Skin Tag Removal

Some essential oils are beneficial in treating skin issues, including skin tags; they are popular because of its antiseptic and antibacterial properties, tea tree essential oil is particularly useful for epidermis/skin issues including pores and skin tags. Tea tree essential oil originates from the Southeast Australian coastline; the essential oil has many health insurance and beauty benefits, including epidermis/skin benefits, dealing with fungal attacks, and clearing coughs and congestion.

Tea tree oil is available for purchase in many big package stores, medication stores, and health food stores. You can even purchase it online. *When buying tea tree essential oil, look for a natural and 100% real oil,* primarily serving as a skin tag removal cream, tea tree oil is effective and natural; however, it will require some time to eliminate your skin tags with tea tree essential oil. *Just how much time depends upon the rate of recurrence of using tea tree essential oil on pores and skin tags and how big is the skin tag.*

For many people, it will require about 14 days before noticing a noticeable difference.

How to Remove Pores and Skin Tags With Tea Tree Oil

There are many solutions to try when working with tea tree oil to eliminate skin tags; a few of them involve combining tea tree essential oil with other natural powerhouses like *apple cider vinegar*.

- Thoroughly clean your skin tag and the area surrounding it.

- Soak a cotton ball and water, squeezing to wring out excess water. Add three drops of tea tree essential oil.

- Apply on the affected epidermis/skin by massaging the cotton softly over the region for five minutes.

- Wash gently with water and pat dried out.

- Continue doing this process three times each day

until the tag falls off.

Ways to get past Skin Tags using Tea Tree Essential oil and Apple Cider Vinegar

- In a little bowl mix collectively four drops of top quality apple cider vinegar, five drops of fresh lemon juice, and three drops of tea tree oil. Blend until thoroughly mixed.

- Drop a cotton ball in this blend then put it on the skin tag.

- Maintain the cotton ball to the pores and skin tag for three to five 5 minutes.

- Wash and pat dry out.

- Continue doing this twice per day for approximately ten times or before the tag falls off.

Ways to get past Skin Tags with Tea Tree Essential oil and Carrier Natural oils

- Combine three drops of tea tree essential oil with any 1 tsp of any carrier essential oil like essential olive oil, coconut essential oil, or jojoba essential oil. If you combine it with coconut essential oil, it will are more of an epidermis/skin tag removal cream because of the coconut oil's regularity.

- Drop a cotton ball into the combination and connect with the affected area by massaging it gently for a few minutes.

- Wash and pat dry out.

- Continue doing this process before the skin tag falls off.

Benefits of Using Tea Tree Essential oil to Remove Epidermis/skin Tags

Tea tree oil is usually safe to use; even women that are pregnant and older people may use it, so long as a health care provider certifies it first. It's an all-natural skin tag removal solution; the procedure is practically pain-free.

Disadvantages of Using Tea Tree Essential oil to Remove Pores and skin Tags

It takes much longer to work than other methods, although it's somewhat frustrating because you have to carry the essential oil onto the region for a few moments during each program, and you ought to apply the necessary oil many times per day.

METHOD #4: Scrape the Skin Tag Off

This technique may be the very best solution to remove skin tags; nevertheless, you should not do that method at home. Trimming or scratching your skin tag off yourself is dangerous, and it leaves you vulnerable to infections, and if done improperly can cause extreme bleeding. If you're interested in using pores and skin tag cut off, see a medical expert to do the task safely.

When to See a medical expert for Epidermis/skin Tag Removal

Though lots of the home cures work wonders to eliminate skin tags, sometimes you should seek a doctor's look after safe skin tag removal. You should visit your skin doctor for pores and skin tag if:

Your skin tag is new: You should have a health care provider check any further development on your skin layer before dealing with it at home. If you don't, you might be inappropriately coping with something much more severe like skin malignancy at home without knowing it.

Your skin tag is sore or red: These may indicate your skin tag is contaminated. Picking at an epidermis/skin tag makes it vulnerable to bacteria and bacterias that can cause infections. If your skin tag shows indicators of an infection, including pain, bloating, redness, or if it's warm or hot touch, see a medical expert at the earliest opportunity.

At home, pores and skin tag removal methods didn't work: Some epidermis/skin tags may be especially stubborn to eliminate at home. When you have attempted at-home removal methods, and your skin tag remains, see a medical expert to help remove it for you.

Your skin tag is within a sensitive area: Pores and skin tags can develop in very delicate areas like close to the groin and on the eyelids. When you have pores and skin tag in either of these places, don't wreak havoc on it yourself; those areas are susceptible and need a doctor's attention for removal.

Your skin tag is significant: Removing a considerable skin tag could cause excess bleeding.

You have specific medical ailments: Some individuals with blood loss disorders and other medical illnesses should never make an effort to the ways to get rid of pores and skin tags at-home methods; doing this might lead to a severe loss of blood. When you have a blood loss disorder or are taking an anticoagulant, see a medical expert to treat your skin layer tags.

What things to Expect Whenever a Doctor Removes a Pores and skin Tag

If you are in none of the situations mentioned previously, you will need a doctor to help you with epidermis/skin tag removal, you might be just a little nervous about the task. Knowing what to expect about how to eliminate pores and skin tags at a doctor's visit can simplify your worries and relax your nerves.

Removing pores and skin tags can be carried out quickly in a dermatologist's office: More often than not, the appointment starts with the skin doctor inspecting your skin tag to be sure that it's only a harmless skin tag. Likely, the skin doctor is also ruling out any indications of contamination as well; from then on the dermatologist will most likely clean the region and use one of the next procedures to eliminate your skin layer tags:

Cutting your skin tag off: Most doctors choose to remove an epidermis/skin tag by slicing it off quickly in the office. The task will start with cleaning the region with an antiseptic solution; concerning the size and located area of the epidermis/skin tag, the physician may rub a numbing solution on your skin layer. Then, the physician uses a very sharpened tool to cut the tag away. The region will be rewashed, and a bandage will be employed. You will probably feel hardly any pain through the process. Most only feel a pinprick feeling; tag removal may necessitate the physician to stitch the producing wound.

Freezing your skin tag: Sometimes, a skin doctor will choose to eliminate a skin tag through freezing it off with very chilly liquid nitrogen. In this technique, the skin doctor cleans the region first and applies numbing cream. Then your dermatologist will swab or aerosol a little amount of water nitrogen in the region. The region may tingle or burn off slightly. Your skin tag should fall off in 10 to 2 weeks.

Burning your skin tag: If reducing or freezing the tag off isn't a choice, the skin doctor may burn your skin tag off. Your skin tag and the encircling area will be washed; the physician then uses a little piece of cable that is warmed with a power current to burn off the stalk of the tag. The heat can help prevent the pores and skin tag from blood loss; the tag should fall off following a procedure.

More often than not, epidermis/skin tag removal causes hardly any bleeding. However, if you undertake bleed carrying out pores and skin tag removal treatment, the physician may apply the cream to avoid the blood loss prior to the area.

Remember, though pores and skin tags can be annoying and unsightly, the majority of time they aren't considered a medical concern, just an aesthetic one. Having said that if you opt to have a health care provider, remove your skin layer tag, consult your insurance provider first. Many won't cover cosmetic epidermis/skin tag removal.

CPSIA information can be obtained
at www.ICGtesting.com
Printed in the USA
BVHW041641120321
602399BV00009B/561